©

Copyright 2022 - All rights reserved.

You may not reproduce, duplicate or send the contents of this book without direct written permission from the author. You cannot apply hereby despite any circumstance blame the publisher or hold him or her to legal responsibility for any reparation, compensations, or monetary forfeiture owing to the information included herein, either in a direct or an indirect way.

Legal Notice: This book has copyright protection. You can use the book for personal purposes. You should not sell, use, alter, distribute, quote, take excerpts, or paraphrase in part or whole the material contained in this book without obtaining the permission of the author first.

Disclaimer Notice: You must take note that the information in this document is for casual reading and entertainment purposes only. We have made every attempt to provide accurate, up-to-date, and reliable information. We do not express or imply guarantees of any kind. The persons who read admit that the writer is not occupied in giving legal, financial, medical, or other advice. We put this book content by sourcing various places.

Please consult a licensed professional before you try any techniques shown in this book. By going through this document, the book lover comes to an an agreement that under no situation is the author accountable for any forfeiture, direct or indirect, which they may incur because of the use of material contained in this document, including, but not limited to, — errors, omissions, or inaccuracies.

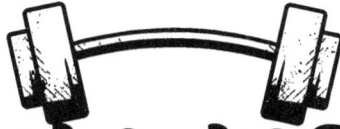

Weight Lifting
Log Book

Belongs to

_____
_____
_____

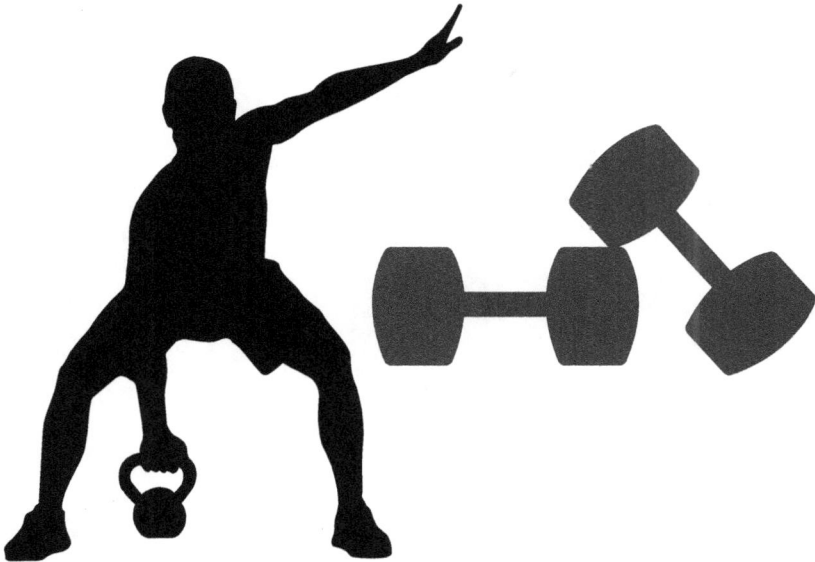

Date:_____   Muscle Group: _____

S M T W T F S   Start Time_____
◯ ◯ ◯ ◯ ◯ ◯ ◯

Weight:_____   Finish Time_____

☐ Upper Body   ☐ Lower Body   ☐ Abs

Exercise	Set	1	2	3	4	5	6	7
	Reps							
	Weight							
	Reps							
	Weight							
	Reps							
	Weight							
	Reps							
	Weight							
	Reps							
	Weight							
	Reps							
	Weight							
	Reps							
	Weight							
	Reps							
	Weight							

Cardio	Time	Distance	Heart Rate	Cals Burned

Measurements

Neck	R Bicep	L Bicep	Chest	Waist	Hips	R Thigh	L Thigh	Calf

Date:_____ Muscle Group: _____

S M T W T F S
○ ○ ○ ○ ○ ○ ○

Start Time_____

Weight:_____ Finish Time_____

☐ Upper Body   ☐ Lower Body   ☐ Abs

Exercise	Set	1	2	3	4	5	6	7
	Reps							
	Weight							
	Reps							
	Weight							
	Reps							
	Weight							
	Reps							
	Weight							
	Reps							
	Weight							
	Reps							
	Weight							
	Reps							
	Weight							
	Reps							
	Weight							

Cardio	Time	Distance	Heart Rate	Cals Burned

Measurements

Neck	R Bicep	L Bicep	Chest	Waist	Hips	R Thigh	L Thigh	Calf

Date:_____ Muscle Group: _____

S M T W T F S   Start Time_____
○ ○ ○ ○ ○ ○ ○

Weight:_____   Finish Time_____

☐ Upper Body   ☐ Lower Body   ☐ Abs

Exercise	Set	1	2	3	4	5	6	7
	Reps							
	Weight							
	Reps							
	Weight							
	Reps							
	Weight							
	Reps							
	Weight							
	Reps							
	Weight							
	Reps							
	Weight							
	Reps							
	Weight							
	Reps							
	Weight							

Cardio	Time	Distance	Heart Rate	Cals Burned

Measurements

Neck	R Bicep	L Bicep	Chest	Waist	Hips	R Thigh	L Thigh	Calf

Date:_____ Muscle Group: _____

S M T W T F S Start Time_____
◯ ◯ ◯ ◯ ◯ ◯ ◯

Weight:_____ Finish Time_____

☐ Upper Body   ☐ Lower Body   ☐ Abs

Exercise	Set	1	2	3	4	5	6	7
	Reps							
	Weight							
	Reps							
	Weight							
	Reps							
	Weight							
	Reps							
	Weight							
	Reps							
	Weight							
	Reps							
	Weight							
	Reps							
	Weight							
	Reps							
	Weight							

Cardio	Time	Distance	Heart Rate	Cals Burned

Measurements

Neck	R Bicep	L Bicep	Chest	Waist	Hips	R Thigh	L Thigh	Calf

Date: _____ **Muscle Group:** _____

S	M	T	W	T	F	S
◯	◯	◯	◯	◯	◯	◯

Start Time _____

Weight: _____ **Finish Time** _____

☐ Upper Body ☐ Lower Body ☐ Abs

Exercise	Set	1	2	3	4	5	6	7
	Reps							
	Weight							
	Reps							
	Weight							
	Reps							
	Weight							
	Reps							
	Weight							
	Reps							
	Weight							
	Reps							
	Weight							
	Reps							
	Weight							
	Reps							
	Weight							

Cardio	Time	Distance	Heart Rate	Cals Burned

Measurements

Neck	R Bicep	L Bicep	Chest	Waist	Hips	R Thigh	L Thigh	Calf

Date:_____ **Muscle Group:** _____

S	M	T	W	T	F	S
○	○	○	○	○	○	○

Start Time_____

Weight:_____ **Finish Time**_____

☐ **Upper Body**   ☐ **Lower Body**   ☐ **Abs**

Exercise	Set	1	2	3	4	5	6	7
	Reps							
	Weight							
	Reps							
	Weight							
	Reps							
	Weight							
	Reps							
	Weight							
	Reps							
	Weight							
	Reps							
	Weight							
	Reps							
	Weight							
	Reps							
	Weight							

Cardio	Time	Distance	Heart Rate	Cals Burned

Measurements

Neck	R Bicep	L Bicep	Chest	Waist	Hips	R Thigh	L Thigh	Calf

Date:_____ **Muscle Group:** _____

S M T W T F S   **Start Time**_____
◯ ◯ ◯ ◯ ◯ ◯ ◯

Weight:_____ **Finish Time**_____

☐ **Upper Body**   ☐ **Lower Body**   ☐ **Abs**

Exercise	Set	1	2	3	4	5	6	7
	Reps							
	Weight							
	Reps							
	Weight							
	Reps							
	Weight							
	Reps							
	Weight							
	Reps							
	Weight							
	Reps							
	Weight							
	Reps							
	Weight							
	Reps							
	Weight							

Cardio	Time	Distance	Heart Rate	Cals Burned

Measurements

Neck	R Bicep	L Bicep	Chest	Waist	Hips	R Thigh	L Thigh	Calf

Date:_____   **Muscle Group:** _____

S	M	T	W	T	F	S
◯	◯	◯	◯	◯	◯	◯

Start Time_____

Weight:_____   **Finish Time**_____

☐ **Upper Body**   ☐ **Lower Body**   ☐ **Abs**

Exercise	Set	1	2	3	4	5	6	7
	Reps							
	Weight							
	Reps							
	Weight							
	Reps							
	Weight							
	Reps							
	Weight							
	Reps							
	Weight							
	Reps							
	Weight							
	Reps							
	Weight							
	Reps							
	Weight							

Cardio	Time	Distance	Heart Rate	Cals Burned

Measurements

Neck	R Bicep	L Bicep	Chest	Waist	Hips	R Thigh	L Thigh	Calf

Date:_____ **Muscle Group:** _____

S M T W T F S **Start Time**_____
◯ ◯ ◯ ◯ ◯ ◯ ◯

Weight:_____ **Finish Time**_____

☐ Upper Body   ☐ Lower Body   ☐ Abs

Exercise	Set	1	2	3	4	5	6	7
	Reps							
	Weight							
	Reps							
	Weight							
	Reps							
	Weight							
	Reps							
	Weight							
	Reps							
	Weight							
	Reps							
	Weight							
	Reps							
	Weight							
	Reps							
	Weight							

Cardio	Time	Distance	Heart Rate	Cals Burned

Measurements

Neck	R Bicep	L Bicep	Chest	Waist	Hips	R Thigh	L Thigh	Calf

Date:_____ **Muscle Group:** _____

S	M	T	W	T	F	S
○	○	○	○	○	○	○

Start Time_____

Weight:_____ **Finish Time**_____

☐ Upper Body ☐ Lower Body ☐ Abs

Exercise	Set	1	2	3	4	5	6	7
	Reps							
	Weight							
	Reps							
	Weight							
	Reps							
	Weight							
	Reps							
	Weight							
	Reps							
	Weight							
	Reps							
	Weight							
	Reps							
	Weight							
	Reps							
	Weight							

Cardio	Time	Distance	Heart Rate	Cals Burned

Measurements

Neck	R Bicep	L Bicep	Chest	Waist	Hips	R Thigh	L Thigh	Calf

Date:_____ **Muscle Group:** _____

S	M	T	W	T	F	S
◯	◯	◯	◯	◯	◯	◯

Start Time_____

Weight:_____ **Finish Time**_____

☐ **Upper Body**   ☐ **Lower Body**   ☐ **Abs**

Exercise	Set	1	2	3	4	5	6	7
	Reps							
	Weight							
	Reps							
	Weight							
	Reps							
	Weight							
	Reps							
	Weight							
	Reps							
	Weight							
	Reps							
	Weight							
	Reps							
	Weight							
	Reps							
	Weight							

Cardio	Time	Distance	Heart Rate	Cals Burned

Measurements

Neck	R Bicep	L Bicep	Chest	Waist	Hips	R Thigh	L Thigh	Calf

Date:_____ Muscle Group: _____

S M T W T F S Start Time_____
◯ ◯ ◯ ◯ ◯ ◯ ◯

Weight:_____ Finish Time_____

☐ Upper Body   ☐ Lower Body   ☐ Abs

Exercise	Set	1	2	3	4	5	6	7
	Reps							
	Weight							
	Reps							
	Weight							
	Reps							
	Weight							
	Reps							
	Weight							
	Reps							
	Weight							
	Reps							
	Weight							
	Reps							
	Weight							
	Reps							
	Weight							

Cardio	Time	Distance	Heart Rate	Cals Burned

Measurements

Neck	R Bicep	L Bicep	Chest	Waist	Hips	R Thigh	L Thigh	Calf

Date:_____   Muscle Group: _____

S M T W T F S   Start Time_____
○ ○ ○ ○ ○ ○ ○

Weight:_____   Finish Time_____

☐ Upper Body   ☐ Lower Body   ☐ Abs

Exercise	Set	1	2	3	4	5	6	7
	Reps							
	Weight							
	Reps							
	Weight							
	Reps							
	Weight							
	Reps							
	Weight							
	Reps							
	Weight							
	Reps							
	Weight							
	Reps							
	Weight							
	Reps							
	Weight							

Cardio	Time	Distance	Heart Rate	Cals Burned

Measurements

Neck	R Bicep	L Bicep	Chest	Waist	Hips	R Thigh	L Thigh	Calf

Date:_____   **Muscle Group:** _____

S   M   T   W   T   F   S   **Start Time**_____

◯ ◯ ◯ ◯ ◯ ◯ ◯

Weight:_____   **Finish Time**_____

☐ **Upper Body**   ☐ **Lower Body**   ☐ **Abs**

Exercise	Set	1	2	3	4	5	6	7
	Reps							
	Weight							
	Reps							
	Weight							
	Reps							
	Weight							
	Reps							
	Weight							
	Reps							
	Weight							
	Reps							
	Weight							
	Reps							
	Weight							
	Reps							
	Weight							

Cardio	Time	Distance	Heart Rate	Cals Burned

Measurements

Neck	R Bicep	L Bicep	Chest	Waist	Hips	R Thigh	L Thigh	Calf

Date:＿＿＿＿＿＿＿ **Muscle Group:** ＿＿＿＿＿＿＿

S M T W T F S **Start Time**＿＿＿＿＿＿＿
○ ○ ○ ○ ○ ○ ○

Weight:＿＿＿＿＿＿＿ **Finish Time**＿＿＿＿＿＿＿

☐ **Upper Body**   ☐ **Lower Body**   ☐ **Abs**

Exercise	Set	1	2	3	4	5	6	7
	Reps							
	Weight							
	Reps							
	Weight							
	Reps							
	Weight							
	Reps							
	Weight							
	Reps							
	Weight							
	Reps							
	Weight							
	Reps							
	Weight							
	Reps							
	Weight							

Cardio	Time	Distance	Heart Rate	Cals Burned

Measurements

Neck	R Bicep	L Bicep	Chest	Waist	Hips	R Thigh	L Thigh	Calf

Date:_____ **Muscle Group:** _____

S M T W T F S   **Start Time**_____
○ ○ ○ ○ ○ ○ ○

Weight:_____   **Finish Time**_____

☐ **Upper Body**   ☐ **Lower Body**   ☐ **Abs**

Exercise	Set	1	2	3	4	5	6	7
	Reps							
	Weight							
	Reps							
	Weight							
	Reps							
	Weight							
	Reps							
	Weight							
	Reps							
	Weight							
	Reps							
	Weight							
	Reps							
	Weight							
	Reps							
	Weight							

Cardio	Time	Distance	Heart Rate	Cals Burned

Measurements

Neck	R Bicep	L Bicep	Chest	Waist	Hips	R Thigh	L Thigh	Calf

Date:_____ **Muscle Group:** _____

S M T W T F S
○ ○ ○ ○ ○ ○ ○

Start Time_____

Weight:_____ **Finish Time**_____

☐ **Upper Body** ☐ **Lower Body** ☐ **Abs**

Exercise	Set	1	2	3	4	5	6	7
	Reps							
	Weight							
	Reps							
	Weight							
	Reps							
	Weight							
	Reps							
	Weight							
	Reps							
	Weight							
	Reps							
	Weight							
	Reps							
	Weight							
	Reps							
	Weight							

Cardio	Time	Distance	Heart Rate	Cals Burned

Measurements

Neck	R Bicep	L Bicep	Chest	Waist	Hips	R Thigh	L Thigh	Calf

Date:_____ Muscle Group: _____

S M T W T F S Start Time_____
○ ○ ○ ○ ○ ○ ○

Weight:_____ Finish Time_____

☐ Upper Body ☐ Lower Body ☐ Abs

Exercise	Set	1	2	3	4	5	6	7
	Reps							
	Weight							
	Reps							
	Weight							
	Reps							
	Weight							
	Reps							
	Weight							
	Reps							
	Weight							
	Reps							
	Weight							
	Reps							
	Weight							
	Reps							
	Weight							

Cardio	Time	Distance	Heart Rate	Cals Burned

Measurements

Neck	R Bicep	L Bicep	Chest	Waist	Hips	R Thigh	L Thigh	Calf

Date: _____   **Muscle Group:** _____

S	M	T	W	T	F	S
◯	◯	◯	◯	◯	◯	◯

Start Time _____

Weight: _____   **Finish Time** _____

☐ Upper Body   ☐ Lower Body   ☐ Abs

Exercise	Set	1	2	3	4	5	6	7
	Reps							
	Weight							
	Reps							
	Weight							
	Reps							
	Weight							
	Reps							
	Weight							
	Reps							
	Weight							
	Reps							
	Weight							
	Reps							
	Weight							
	Reps							
	Weight							

Cardio	Time	Distance	Heart Rate	Cals Burned

Measurements

Neck	R Bicep	L Bicep	Chest	Waist	Hips	R Thigh	L Thigh	Calf

Date:_____ Muscle Group: _____

S M T W T F S   Start Time_____
◯ ◯ ◯ ◯ ◯ ◯ ◯

Weight:_____   Finish Time_____

☐ Upper Body   ☐ Lower Body   ☐ Abs

Exercise	Set	1	2	3	4	5	6	7
	Reps							
	Weight							
	Reps							
	Weight							
	Reps							
	Weight							
	Reps							
	Weight							
	Reps							
	Weight							
	Reps							
	Weight							
	Reps							
	Weight							
	Reps							
	Weight							

Cardio	Time	Distance	Heart Rate	Cals Burned

Measurements

Neck	R Bicep	L Bicep	Chest	Waist	Hips	R Thigh	L Thigh	Calf

Date:_____ **Muscle Group:** _____

S	M	T	W	T	F	S
○	○	○	○	○	○	○

Start Time_____

Weight:_____ **Finish Time**_____

☐ Upper Body   ☐ Lower Body   ☐ Abs

Exercise	Set	1	2	3	4	5	6	7
	Reps							
	Weight							
	Reps							
	Weight							
	Reps							
	Weight							
	Reps							
	Weight							
	Reps							
	Weight							
	Reps							
	Weight							
	Reps							
	Weight							
	Reps							
	Weight							

Cardio	Time	Distance	Heart Rate	Cals Burned

Measurements

Neck	R Bicep	L Bicep	Chest	Waist	Hips	R Thigh	L Thigh	Calf

Date:_____ **Muscle Group:** _____

S	M	T	W	T	F	S
◯	◯	◯	◯	◯	◯	◯

Start Time _____

Weight:_____ **Finish Time** _____

☐ **Upper Body**　　☐ **Lower Body**　　☐ **Abs**

Exercise	Set	1	2	3	4	5	6	7
	Reps							
	Weight							
	Reps							
	Weight							
	Reps							
	Weight							
	Reps							
	Weight							
	Reps							
	Weight							
	Reps							
	Weight							
	Reps							
	Weight							
	Reps							
	Weight							

Cardio	Time	Distance	Heart Rate	Cals Burned

Measurements

Neck	R Bicep	L Bicep	Chest	Waist	Hips	R Thigh	L Thigh	Calf

Date:_____ Muscle Group: _____

S M T W T F S   Start Time_____
◯ ◯ ◯ ◯ ◯ ◯ ◯

Weight:_____ Finish Time_____

☐ Upper Body   ☐ Lower Body   ☐ Abs

Exercise	Set	1	2	3	4	5	6	7
	Reps							
	Weight							
	Reps							
	Weight							
	Reps							
	Weight							
	Reps							
	Weight							
	Reps							
	Weight							
	Reps							
	Weight							
	Reps							
	Weight							
	Reps							
	Weight							

Cardio	Time	Distance	Heart Rate	Cals Burned

Measurements

Neck	R Bicep	L Bicep	Chest	Waist	Hips	R Thigh	L Thigh	Calf

Date:_____ **Muscle Group:** _____

S M T W T F S **Start Time**_____
○ ○ ○ ○ ○ ○ ○

Weight:_____ **Finish Time**_____

☐ **Upper Body**   ☐ **Lower Body**   ☐ **Abs**

Exercise	Set	1	2	3	4	5	6	7
	Reps							
	Weight							
	Reps							
	Weight							
	Reps							
	Weight							
	Reps							
	Weight							
	Reps							
	Weight							
	Reps							
	Weight							
	Reps							
	Weight							
	Reps							
	Weight							

Cardio	Time	Distance	Heart Rate	Cals Burned

Measurements

Neck	R Bicep	L Bicep	Chest	Waist	Hips	R Thigh	L Thigh	Calf

Date:_____ Muscle Group: _____

S M T W T F S   Start Time_____
◯ ◯ ◯ ◯ ◯ ◯ ◯

Weight:_____   Finish Time_____

☐ Upper Body   ☐ Lower Body   ☐ Abs

Exercise	Set	1	2	3	4	5	6	7
	Reps							
	Weight							
	Reps							
	Weight							
	Reps							
	Weight							
	Reps							
	Weight							
	Reps							
	Weight							
	Reps							
	Weight							
	Reps							
	Weight							
	Reps							
	Weight							

Cardio	Time	Distance	Heart Rate	Cals Burned

Measurements

Neck	R Bicep	L Bicep	Chest	Waist	Hips	R Thigh	L Thigh	Calf

Date:_____   Muscle Group: _____

S   M   T   W   T   F   S   Start Time_____
◯   ◯   ◯   ◯   ◯   ◯   ◯

Weight:_____   Finish Time_____

☐ Upper Body   ☐ Lower Body   ☐ Abs

Exercise	Set	1	2	3	4	5	6	7
	Reps							
	Weight							
	Reps							
	Weight							
	Reps							
	Weight							
	Reps							
	Weight							
	Reps							
	Weight							
	Reps							
	Weight							
	Reps							
	Weight							
	Reps							
	Weight							

Cardio	Time	Distance	Heart Rate	Cals Burned

Measurements

Neck	R Bicep	L Bicep	Chest	Waist	Hips	R Thigh	L Thigh	Calf

Date:_____ Muscle Group: _____

S M T W T F S   Start Time_____
◯ ◯ ◯ ◯ ◯ ◯ ◯

Weight:_____   Finish Time_____

☐ Upper Body   ☐ Lower Body   ☐ Abs

Exercise	Set	1	2	3	4	5	6	7
	Reps							
	Weight							
	Reps							
	Weight							
	Reps							
	Weight							
	Reps							
	Weight							
	Reps							
	Weight							
	Reps							
	Weight							
	Reps							
	Weight							
	Reps							
	Weight							

Cardio	Time	Distance	Heart Rate	Cals Burned

Measurements

Neck	R Bicep	L Bicep	Chest	Waist	Hips	R Thigh	L Thigh	Calf

Date:_____ Muscle Group: _____

S M T W T F S   Start Time_____
○ ○ ○ ○ ○ ○ ○

Weight:_____   Finish Time_____

☐ Upper Body   ☐ Lower Body   ☐ Abs

Exercise	Set	1	2	3	4	5	6	7
	Reps							
	Weight							
	Reps							
	Weight							
	Reps							
	Weight							
	Reps							
	Weight							
	Reps							
	Weight							
	Reps							
	Weight							
	Reps							
	Weight							
	Reps							
	Weight							

Cardio	Time	Distance	Heart Rate	Cals Burned

Measurements

Neck	R Bicep	L Bicep	Chest	Waist	Hips	R Thigh	L Thigh	Calf

Date:_____ Muscle Group: _____

S M T W T F S   Start Time_____
◯ ◯ ◯ ◯ ◯ ◯ ◯

Weight:_____   Finish Time_____

☐ Upper Body   ☐ Lower Body   ☐ Abs

Exercise	Set	1	2	3	4	5	6	7
	Reps							
	Weight							
	Reps							
	Weight							
	Reps							
	Weight							
	Reps							
	Weight							
	Reps							
	Weight							
	Reps							
	Weight							
	Reps							
	Weight							
	Reps							
	Weight							

Cardio	Time	Distance	Heart Rate	Cals Burned

Measurements

Neck	R Bicep	L Bicep	Chest	Waist	Hips	R Thigh	L Thigh	Calf

Date:_____   **Muscle Group:** _____

S M T W T F S   **Start Time**_____
○ ○ ○ ○ ○ ○ ○

Weight:_____   **Finish Time**_____

☐ **Upper Body**   ☐ **Lower Body**   ☐ **Abs**

Exercise	Set	1	2	3	4	5	6	7
	Reps							
	Weight							
	Reps							
	Weight							
	Reps							
	Weight							
	Reps							
	Weight							
	Reps							
	Weight							
	Reps							
	Weight							
	Reps							
	Weight							
	Reps							
	Weight							

Cardio	Time	Distance	Heart Rate	Cals Burned

Measurements

Neck	R Bicep	L Bicep	Chest	Waist	Hips	R Thigh	L Thigh	Calf

Date:_____   Muscle Group: _____

S   M   T   W   T   F   S   Start Time_____
◯   ◯   ◯   ◯   ◯   ◯   ◯

Weight:_____   Finish Time_____

☐ Upper Body   ☐ Lower Body   ☐ Abs

Exercise	Set	1	2	3	4	5	6	7
	Reps							
	Weight							
	Reps							
	Weight							
	Reps							
	Weight							
	Reps							
	Weight							
	Reps							
	Weight							
	Reps							
	Weight							
	Reps							
	Weight							
	Reps							
	Weight							

Cardio	Time	Distance	Heart Rate	Cals Burned

Measurements

Neck	R Bicep	L Bicep	Chest	Waist	Hips	R Thigh	L Thigh	Calf

Date:_____ **Muscle Group:** _____

S   M   T   W   T   F   S   **Start Time**_____
○   ○   ○   ○   ○   ○   ○

Weight:_____ **Finish Time**_____

☐ **Upper Body**   ☐ **Lower Body**   ☐ **Abs**

Exercise	Set	1	2	3	4	5	6	7
	Reps							
	Weight							
	Reps							
	Weight							
	Reps							
	Weight							
	Reps							
	Weight							
	Reps							
	Weight							
	Reps							
	Weight							
	Reps							
	Weight							
	Reps							
	Weight							

Cardio	Time	Distance	Heart Rate	Cals Burned

Measurements

Neck	R Bicep	L Bicep	Chest	Waist	Hips	R Thigh	L Thigh	Calf

Date:_____ Muscle Group: _____

S M T W T F S   Start Time_____
○ ○ ○ ○ ○ ○ ○

Weight:_____ Finish Time_____

☐ Upper Body   ☐ Lower Body   ☐ Abs

Exercise	Set	1	2	3	4	5	6	7
	Reps							
	Weight							
	Reps							
	Weight							
	Reps							
	Weight							
	Reps							
	Weight							
	Reps							
	Weight							
	Reps							
	Weight							
	Reps							
	Weight							
	Reps							
	Weight							

Cardio	Time	Distance	Heart Rate	Cals Burned

Measurements

Neck	R Bicep	L Bicep	Chest	Waist	Hips	R Thigh	L Thigh	Calf

Date:_____   **Muscle Group:** _____

S   M   T   W   T   F   S   **Start Time**_____
○ ○ ○ ○ ○ ○ ○

Weight:_____   **Finish Time**_____

☐ **Upper Body**   ☐ **Lower Body**   ☐ **Abs**

Exercise	Set	1	2	3	4	5	6	7
	Reps							
	Weight							
	Reps							
	Weight							
	Reps							
	Weight							
	Reps							
	Weight							
	Reps							
	Weight							
	Reps							
	Weight							
	Reps							
	Weight							
	Reps							
	Weight							

Cardio	Time	Distance	Heart Rate	Cals Burned

Measurements

Neck	R Bicep	L Bicep	Chest	Waist	Hips	R Thigh	L Thigh	Calf

Date:_____ Muscle Group: _____

S   M   T   W   T   F   S   Start Time_____
◯ ◯ ◯ ◯ ◯ ◯ ◯

Weight:_____   Finish Time_____

☐ Upper Body   ☐ Lower Body   ☐ Abs

Exercise	Set	1	2	3	4	5	6	7
	Reps							
	Weight							
	Reps							
	Weight							
	Reps							
	Weight							
	Reps							
	Weight							
	Reps							
	Weight							
	Reps							
	Weight							
	Reps							
	Weight							
	Reps							
	Weight							

Cardio	Time	Distance	Heart Rate	Cals Burned

Measurements

Neck	R Bicep	L Bicep	Chest	Waist	Hips	R Thigh	L Thigh	Calf

Date:_____ Muscle Group: _____

S M T W T F S
○ ○ ○ ○ ○ ○ ○

Start Time_____

Weight:_____

Finish Time_____

☐ Upper Body   ☐ Lower Body   ☐ Abs

Exercise	Set	1	2	3	4	5	6	7
	Reps							
	Weight							
	Reps							
	Weight							
	Reps							
	Weight							
	Reps							
	Weight							
	Reps							
	Weight							
	Reps							
	Weight							
	Reps							
	Weight							
	Reps							
	Weight							

Cardio	Time	Distance	Heart Rate	Cals Burned

Measurements

Neck	R Bicep	L Bicep	Chest	Waist	Hips	R Thigh	L Thigh	Calf

Date:_____   Muscle Group: _____

S M T W T F S   Start Time_____
○ ○ ○ ○ ○ ○ ○

Weight:_____   Finish Time_____

☐ Upper Body   ☐ Lower Body   ☐ Abs

Exercise	Set	1	2	3	4	5	6	7
	Reps							
	Weight							
	Reps							
	Weight							
	Reps							
	Weight							
	Reps							
	Weight							
	Reps							
	Weight							
	Reps							
	Weight							
	Reps							
	Weight							
	Reps							
	Weight							

Cardio	Time	Distance	Heart Rate	Cals Burned

Measurements

Neck	R Bicep	L Bicep	Chest	Waist	Hips	R Thigh	L Thigh	Calf

Date:_____   **Muscle Group:** _____

S   M   T   W   T   F   S   **Start Time**_____
◯ ◯ ◯ ◯ ◯ ◯ ◯

Weight:_____   **Finish Time**_____

☐ Upper Body   ☐ Lower Body   ☐ Abs

Exercise	Set	1	2	3	4	5	6	7
	Reps							
	Weight							
	Reps							
	Weight							
	Reps							
	Weight							
	Reps							
	Weight							
	Reps							
	Weight							
	Reps							
	Weight							
	Reps							
	Weight							
	Reps							
	Weight							

Cardio	Time	Distance	Heart Rate	Cals Burned

Measurements

Neck	R Bicep	L Bicep	Chest	Waist	Hips	R Thigh	L Thigh	Calf

Date:_____ **Muscle Group:** _____

S M T W T F S   **Start Time**_____
◯ ◯ ◯ ◯ ◯ ◯ ◯

Weight:_____ **Finish Time**_____

☐ Upper Body   ☐ Lower Body   ☐ Abs

Exercise	Set	1	2	3	4	5	6	7
	Reps							
	Weight							
	Reps							
	Weight							
	Reps							
	Weight							
	Reps							
	Weight							
	Reps							
	Weight							
	Reps							
	Weight							
	Reps							
	Weight							
	Reps							
	Weight							

Cardio	Time	Distance	Heart Rate	Cals Burned

Measurements

Neck	R Bicep	L Bicep	Chest	Waist	Hips	R Thigh	L Thigh	Calf

Date:_____ **Muscle Group:** _____

S M T W T F S   **Start Time**_____
○ ○ ○ ○ ○ ○ ○

Weight:_____ **Finish Time**_____

☐ **Upper Body**   ☐ **Lower Body**   ☐ **Abs**

Exercise	Set	1	2	3	4	5	6	7
	Reps							
	Weight							
	Reps							
	Weight							
	Reps							
	Weight							
	Reps							
	Weight							
	Reps							
	Weight							
	Reps							
	Weight							
	Reps							
	Weight							
	Reps							
	Weight							

Cardio	Time	Distance	Heart Rate	Cals Burned

Measurements

Neck	R Bicep	L Bicep	Chest	Waist	Hips	R Thigh	L Thigh	Calf

Date:_____   **Muscle Group:** _____

S M T W T F S   **Start Time**_____
◯ ◯ ◯ ◯ ◯ ◯ ◯

Weight:_____   **Finish Time**_____

☐ **Upper Body**   ☐ **Lower Body**   ☐ **Abs**

Exercise	Set	1	2	3	4	5	6	7
	Reps							
	Weight							
	Reps							
	Weight							
	Reps							
	Weight							
	Reps							
	Weight							
	Reps							
	Weight							
	Reps							
	Weight							
	Reps							
	Weight							
	Reps							
	Weight							

Cardio	Time	Distance	Heart Rate	Cals Burned

Measurements

Neck	R Bicep	L Bicep	Chest	Waist	Hips	R Thigh	L Thigh	Calf

Date:_____ **Muscle Group:** _____

S M T W T F S **Start Time**_____
○ ○ ○ ○ ○ ○ ○

Weight:_____ **Finish Time**_____

☐ **Upper Body**   ☐ **Lower Body**   ☐ **Abs**

Exercise	Set	1	2	3	4	5	6	7
	Reps							
	Weight							
	Reps							
	Weight							
	Reps							
	Weight							
	Reps							
	Weight							
	Reps							
	Weight							
	Reps							
	Weight							
	Reps							
	Weight							
	Reps							
	Weight							

Cardio	Time	Distance	Heart Rate	Cals Burned

Measurements

Neck	R Bicep	L Bicep	Chest	Waist	Hips	R Thigh	L Thigh	Calf

Date:_____ **Muscle Group:** _____

S M T W T F S   **Start Time**_____
○ ○ ○ ○ ○ ○ ○

Weight:_____   **Finish Time**_____

☐ Upper Body   ☐ Lower Body   ☐ Abs

Exercise	Set	1	2	3	4	5	6	7
	Reps							
	Weight							
	Reps							
	Weight							
	Reps							
	Weight							
	Reps							
	Weight							
	Reps							
	Weight							
	Reps							
	Weight							
	Reps							
	Weight							
	Reps							
	Weight							

Cardio	Time	Distance	Heart Rate	Cals Burned

Measurements

Neck	R Bicep	L Bicep	Chest	Waist	Hips	R Thigh	L Thigh	Calf

Date:_____ Muscle Group: _____

S	M	T	W	T	F	S
◯	◯	◯	◯	◯	◯	◯

Start Time_____

Weight:_____ Finish Time_____

☐ Upper Body ☐ Lower Body ☐ Abs

Exercise	Set	1	2	3	4	5	6	7
	Reps							
	Weight							
	Reps							
	Weight							
	Reps							
	Weight							
	Reps							
	Weight							
	Reps							
	Weight							
	Reps							
	Weight							
	Reps							
	Weight							
	Reps							
	Weight							

Cardio	Time	Distance	Heart Rate	Cals Burned

Measurements

Neck	R Bicep	L Bicep	Chest	Waist	Hips	R Thigh	L Thigh	Calf

Date:_____ Muscle Group: _____

S M T W T F S Start Time_____
◯ ◯ ◯ ◯ ◯ ◯ ◯

Weight:_____ Finish Time_____

☐ Upper Body ☐ Lower Body ☐ Abs

Exercise	Set	1	2	3	4	5	6	7
	Reps							
	Weight							
	Reps							
	Weight							
	Reps							
	Weight							
	Reps							
	Weight							
	Reps							
	Weight							
	Reps							
	Weight							
	Reps							
	Weight							
	Reps							
	Weight							

Cardio	Time	Distance	Heart Rate	Cals Burned

Measurements

Neck	R Bicep	L Bicep	Chest	Waist	Hips	R Thigh	L Thigh	Calf

Date:_____   **Muscle Group:** _____

S	M	T	W	T	F	S
◯	◯	◯	◯	◯	◯	◯

Start Time_____

Weight:_____   **Finish Time**_____

☐ Upper Body   ☐ Lower Body   ☐ Abs

Exercise	Set	1	2	3	4	5	6	7
	Reps							
	Weight							
	Reps							
	Weight							
	Reps							
	Weight							
	Reps							
	Weight							
	Reps							
	Weight							
	Reps							
	Weight							
	Reps							
	Weight							
	Reps							
	Weight							

Cardio	Time	Distance	Heart Rate	Cals Burned

Measurements

Neck	R Bicep	L Bicep	Chest	Waist	Hips	R Thigh	L Thigh	Calf

Date:_____   **Muscle Group:** _____

S   M   T   W   T   F   S   **Start Time**_____
◯ ◯ ◯ ◯ ◯ ◯ ◯

Weight:_____   **Finish Time**_____

☐ Upper Body   ☐ Lower Body   ☐ Abs

Exercise	Set	1	2	3	4	5	6	7
	Reps							
	Weight							
	Reps							
	Weight							
	Reps							
	Weight							
	Reps							
	Weight							
	Reps							
	Weight							
	Reps							
	Weight							
	Reps							
	Weight							
	Reps							
	Weight							

Cardio	Time	Distance	Heart Rate	Cals Burned

Measurements

Neck	R Bicep	L Bicep	Chest	Waist	Hips	R Thigh	L Thigh	Calf

Date:_____ **Muscle Group:** _____

S M T W T F S   **Start Time**_____
◯ ◯ ◯ ◯ ◯ ◯ ◯

Weight:_____ **Finish Time**_____

☐ **Upper Body**   ☐ **Lower Body**   ☐ **Abs**

Exercise	Set	1	2	3	4	5	6	7
	Reps							
	Weight							
	Reps							
	Weight							
	Reps							
	Weight							
	Reps							
	Weight							
	Reps							
	Weight							
	Reps							
	Weight							
	Reps							
	Weight							
	Reps							
	Weight							

Cardio	Time	Distance	Heart Rate	Cals Burned

Measurements

Neck	R Bicep	L Bicep	Chest	Waist	Hips	R Thigh	L Thigh	Calf

Date:_____   Muscle Group: _____

S M T W T F S   Start Time_____
○ ○ ○ ○ ○ ○ ○

Weight:_____   Finish Time_____

☐ Upper Body   ☐ Lower Body   ☐ Abs

Exercise	Set	1	2	3	4	5	6	7
	Reps							
	Weight							
	Reps							
	Weight							
	Reps							
	Weight							
	Reps							
	Weight							
	Reps							
	Weight							
	Reps							
	Weight							
	Reps							
	Weight							
	Reps							
	Weight							

Cardio	Time	Distance	Heart Rate	Cals Burned

Measurements

Neck	R Bicep	L Bicep	Chest	Waist	Hips	R Thigh	L Thigh	Calf

Date:_____ Muscle Group: _____

S M T W T F S   Start Time_____
◯ ◯ ◯ ◯ ◯ ◯ ◯

Weight:_____ Finish Time_____

☐ Upper Body   ☐ Lower Body   ☐ Abs

Exercise	Set	1	2	3	4	5	6	7
	Reps							
	Weight							
	Reps							
	Weight							
	Reps							
	Weight							
	Reps							
	Weight							
	Reps							
	Weight							
	Reps							
	Weight							
	Reps							
	Weight							
	Reps							
	Weight							

Cardio	Time	Distance	Heart Rate	Cals Burned

Measurements

Neck	R Bicep	L Bicep	Chest	Waist	Hips	R Thigh	L Thigh	Calf

Date:_____ Muscle Group: _____

S M T W T F S   **Start Time**_____

◯◯◯◯◯◯◯

Weight:_____   **Finish Time**_____

☐ Upper Body   ☐ Lower Body   ☐ Abs

Exercise	Set	1	2	3	4	5	6	7
	Reps							
	Weight							
	Reps							
	Weight							
	Reps							
	Weight							
	Reps							
	Weight							
	Reps							
	Weight							
	Reps							
	Weight							
	Reps							
	Weight							
	Reps							
	Weight							

Cardio	Time	Distance	Heart Rate	Cals Burned

Measurements

Neck	R Bicep	L Bicep	Chest	Waist	Hips	R Thigh	L Thigh	Calf

Date:_____ **Muscle Group:** _____

S	M	T	W	T	F	S
◯	◯	◯	◯	◯	◯	◯

Start Time_____

Weight:_____ **Finish Time**_____

☐ Upper Body ☐ Lower Body ☐ Abs

Exercise	Set	1	2	3	4	5	6	7
	Reps							
	Weight							
	Reps							
	Weight							
	Reps							
	Weight							
	Reps							
	Weight							
	Reps							
	Weight							
	Reps							
	Weight							
	Reps							
	Weight							
	Reps							
	Weight							

Cardio	Time	Distance	Heart Rate	Cals Burned

Measurements

Neck	R Bicep	L Bicep	Chest	Waist	Hips	R Thigh	L Thigh	Calf

Date:_____ **Muscle Group:** _____

S M T W T F S   **Start Time**_____
○ ○ ○ ○ ○ ○ ○

Weight:_____ **Finish Time**_____

☐ **Upper Body** ☐ **Lower Body** ☐ **Abs**

Exercise	Set	1	2	3	4	5	6	7
	Reps							
	Weight							
	Reps							
	Weight							
	Reps							
	Weight							
	Reps							
	Weight							
	Reps							
	Weight							
	Reps							
	Weight							
	Reps							
	Weight							
	Reps							
	Weight							

Cardio	Time	Distance	Heart Rate	Cals Burned

Measurements

Neck	R Bicep	L Bicep	Chest	Waist	Hips	R Thigh	L Thigh	Calf

Date:_____ Muscle Group: _____

S M T W T F S   Start Time_____
◯ ◯ ◯ ◯ ◯ ◯ ◯

Weight:_____   Finish Time_____

☐ Upper Body   ☐ Lower Body   ☐ Abs

Exercise	Set	1	2	3	4	5	6	7
	Reps							
	Weight							
	Reps							
	Weight							
	Reps							
	Weight							
	Reps							
	Weight							
	Reps							
	Weight							
	Reps							
	Weight							
	Reps							
	Weight							
	Reps							
	Weight							

Cardio	Time	Distance	Heart Rate	Cals Burned

Measurements

Neck	R Bicep	L Bicep	Chest	Waist	Hips	R Thigh	L Thigh	Calf

Date:_____ Muscle Group: _____

S	M	T	W	T	F	S
◯	◯	◯	◯	◯	◯	◯

Start Time_____

Weight:_____ **Finish Time**_____

☐ Upper Body ☐ Lower Body ☐ Abs

Exercise	Set	1	2	3	4	5	6	7
	Reps							
	Weight							
	Reps							
	Weight							
	Reps							
	Weight							
	Reps							
	Weight							
	Reps							
	Weight							
	Reps							
	Weight							
	Reps							
	Weight							
	Reps							
	Weight							

Cardio	Time	Distance	Heart Rate	Cals Burned

Measurements

Neck	R Bicep	L Bicep	Chest	Waist	Hips	R Thigh	L Thigh	Calf

Date:_____ **Muscle Group:** _____

S M T W T F S   **Start Time**_____
◯ ◯ ◯ ◯ ◯ ◯ ◯

Weight:_____   **Finish Time**_____

☐ **Upper Body**   ☐ **Lower Body**   ☐ **Abs**

Exercise	Set	1	2	3	4	5	6	7
	Reps							
	Weight							
	Reps							
	Weight							
	Reps							
	Weight							
	Reps							
	Weight							
	Reps							
	Weight							
	Reps							
	Weight							
	Reps							
	Weight							
	Reps							
	Weight							

Cardio	Time	Distance	Heart Rate	Cals Burned

Measurements

Neck	R Bicep	L Bicep	Chest	Waist	Hips	R Thigh	L Thigh	Calf

Date:_____ Muscle Group: _____

S   M   T   W   T   F   S   Start Time_____
◯ ◯ ◯ ◯ ◯ ◯ ◯

Weight:_____   Finish Time_____

☐ Upper Body   ☐ Lower Body   ☐ Abs

Exercise	Set	1	2	3	4	5	6	7
	Reps							
	Weight							
	Reps							
	Weight							
	Reps							
	Weight							
	Reps							
	Weight							
	Reps							
	Weight							
	Reps							
	Weight							
	Reps							
	Weight							
	Reps							
	Weight							

Cardio	Time	Distance	Heart Rate	Cals Burned

Measurements

Neck	R Bicep	L Bicep	Chest	Waist	Hips	R Thigh	L Thigh	Calf

Date:_____ Muscle Group: _____

S M T W T F S   Start Time_____
◯ ◯ ◯ ◯ ◯ ◯ ◯

Weight:_____   Finish Time_____

☐ Upper Body   ☐ Lower Body   ☐ Abs

Exercise	Set	1	2	3	4	5	6	7
	Reps							
	Weight							
	Reps							
	Weight							
	Reps							
	Weight							
	Reps							
	Weight							
	Reps							
	Weight							
	Reps							
	Weight							
	Reps							
	Weight							
	Reps							
	Weight							

Cardio	Time	Distance	Heart Rate	Cals Burned

Measurements

Neck	R Bicep	L Bicep	Chest	Waist	Hips	R Thigh	L Thigh	Calf

Date:_____ Muscle Group: _____

S M T W T F S   Start Time_____
○ ○ ○ ○ ○ ○ ○

Weight:_____ Finish Time_____

☐ Upper Body   ☐ Lower Body   ☐ Abs

Exercise	Set	1	2	3	4	5	6	7
	Reps							
	Weight							
	Reps							
	Weight							
	Reps							
	Weight							
	Reps							
	Weight							
	Reps							
	Weight							
	Reps							
	Weight							
	Reps							
	Weight							
	Reps							
	Weight							

Cardio	Time	Distance	Heart Rate	Cals Burned

Measurements

Neck	R Bicep	L Bicep	Chest	Waist	Hips	R Thigh	L Thigh	Calf

Date:_____ **Muscle Group:** _____

S	M	T	W	T	F	S
○	○	○	○	○	○	○

Start Time_____

Weight:_____ **Finish Time**_____

☐ **Upper Body**   ☐ **Lower Body**   ☐ **Abs**

Exercise	Set	1	2	3	4	5	6	7
	Reps							
	Weight							
	Reps							
	Weight							
	Reps							
	Weight							
	Reps							
	Weight							
	Reps							
	Weight							
	Reps							
	Weight							
	Reps							
	Weight							
	Reps							
	Weight							

Cardio	Time	Distance	Heart Rate	Cals Burned

Measurements

Neck	R Bicep	L Bicep	Chest	Waist	Hips	R Thigh	L Thigh	Calf

Date:_____   Muscle Group: _____

S M T W T F S   Start Time_____
○ ○ ○ ○ ○ ○ ○

Weight:_____   Finish Time_____

☐ Upper Body   ☐ Lower Body   ☐ Abs

Exercise	Set	1	2	3	4	5	6	7
	Reps							
	Weight							
	Reps							
	Weight							
	Reps							
	Weight							
	Reps							
	Weight							
	Reps							
	Weight							
	Reps							
	Weight							
	Reps							
	Weight							
	Reps							
	Weight							

Cardio	Time	Distance	Heart Rate	Cals Burned

Measurements

Neck	R Bicep	L Bicep	Chest	Waist	Hips	R Thigh	L Thigh	Calf

Date:_____ Muscle Group: _____

S M T W T F S   Start Time_____
○ ○ ○ ○ ○ ○ ○

Weight:_____   Finish Time_____

☐ Upper Body   ☐ Lower Body   ☐ Abs

Exercise	Set	1	2	3	4	5	6	7
	Reps							
	Weight							
	Reps							
	Weight							
	Reps							
	Weight							
	Reps							
	Weight							
	Reps							
	Weight							
	Reps							
	Weight							
	Reps							
	Weight							
	Reps							
	Weight							

Cardio	Time	Distance	Heart Rate	Cals Burned

Measurements

Neck	R Bicep	L Bicep	Chest	Waist	Hips	R Thigh	L Thigh	Calf

Date:_____ Muscle Group: _____

S M T W T F S Start Time_____
◯ ◯ ◯ ◯ ◯ ◯ ◯

Weight:_____ Finish Time_____

☐ Upper Body ☐ Lower Body ☐ Abs

Exercise	Set	1	2	3	4	5	6	7
	Reps							
	Weight							
	Reps							
	Weight							
	Reps							
	Weight							
	Reps							
	Weight							
	Reps							
	Weight							
	Reps							
	Weight							
	Reps							
	Weight							
	Reps							
	Weight							

Cardio	Time	Distance	Heart Rate	Cals Burned

Measurements

Neck	R Bicep	L Bicep	Chest	Waist	Hips	R Thigh	L Thigh	Calf

Date:_____   **Muscle Group:** _____

S	M	T	W	T	F	S
◯	◯	◯	◯	◯	◯	◯

Start Time_____

Weight:_____   **Finish Time**_____

☐ **Upper Body**   ☐ **Lower Body**   ☐ **Abs**

Exercise	Set	1	2	3	4	5	6	7
	Reps							
	Weight							
	Reps							
	Weight							
	Reps							
	Weight							
	Reps							
	Weight							
	Reps							
	Weight							
	Reps							
	Weight							
	Reps							
	Weight							
	Reps							
	Weight							

Cardio	Time	Distance	Heart Rate	Cals Burned

Measurements

Neck	R Bicep	L Bicep	Chest	Waist	Hips	R Thigh	L Thigh	Calf

Date:_____ **Muscle Group:** _____

S M T W T F S
◯ ◯ ◯ ◯ ◯ ◯ ◯

Start Time_____

Weight:_____

Finish Time_____

☐ **Upper Body**   ☐ **Lower Body**   ☐ **Abs**

Exercise	Set	1	2	3	4	5	6	7
	Reps							
	Weight							
	Reps							
	Weight							
	Reps							
	Weight							
	Reps							
	Weight							
	Reps							
	Weight							
	Reps							
	Weight							
	Reps							
	Weight							
	Reps							
	Weight							

Cardio	Time	Distance	Heart Rate	Cals Burned

Measurements

Neck	R Bicep	L Bicep	Chest	Waist	Hips	R Thigh	L Thigh	Calf

Date:_____   **Muscle Group:** _____

S M T W T F S   **Start Time**_____
◯ ◯ ◯ ◯ ◯ ◯ ◯

Weight:_____   **Finish Time**_____

☐ **Upper Body**   ☐ **Lower Body**   ☐ **Abs**

Exercise	Set	1	2	3	4	5	6	7
	Reps							
	Weight							
	Reps							
	Weight							
	Reps							
	Weight							
	Reps							
	Weight							
	Reps							
	Weight							
	Reps							
	Weight							
	Reps							
	Weight							
	Reps							
	Weight							

Cardio	Time	Distance	Heart Rate	Cals Burned

Measurements

Neck	R Bicep	L Bicep	Chest	Waist	Hips	R Thigh	L Thigh	Calf

Date:_____ **Muscle Group:** _____

S	M	T	W	T	F	S
○	○	○	○	○	○	○

Start Time_____

Weight:_____ **Finish Time**_____

☐ Upper Body   ☐ Lower Body   ☐ Abs

Exercise	Set	1	2	3	4	5	6	7
	Reps							
	Weight							
	Reps							
	Weight							
	Reps							
	Weight							
	Reps							
	Weight							
	Reps							
	Weight							
	Reps							
	Weight							
	Reps							
	Weight							
	Reps							
	Weight							

Cardio	Time	Distance	Heart Rate	Cals Burned

Measurements

Neck	R Bicep	L Bicep	Chest	Waist	Hips	R Thigh	L Thigh	Calf

Date:_____ **Muscle Group:** _____

S M T W T F S   **Start Time**_____
◯ ◯ ◯ ◯ ◯ ◯ ◯

Weight:_____   **Finish Time**_____

☐ **Upper Body**   ☐ **Lower Body**   ☐ **Abs**

Exercise	Set	1	2	3	4	5	6	7
	Reps							
	Weight							
	Reps							
	Weight							
	Reps							
	Weight							
	Reps							
	Weight							
	Reps							
	Weight							
	Reps							
	Weight							
	Reps							
	Weight							
	Reps							
	Weight							

Cardio	Time	Distance	Heart Rate	Cals Burned

Measurements

Neck	R Bicep	L Bicep	Chest	Waist	Hips	R Thigh	L Thigh	Calf

Date:_____ **Muscle Group:** _____

S M T W T F S   **Start Time**_____
◯ ◯ ◯ ◯ ◯ ◯ ◯

Weight:_____ **Finish Time**_____

☐ **Upper Body**   ☐ **Lower Body**   ☐ **Abs**

Exercise	Set	1	2	3	4	5	6	7
	Reps							
	Weight							
	Reps							
	Weight							
	Reps							
	Weight							
	Reps							
	Weight							
	Reps							
	Weight							
	Reps							
	Weight							
	Reps							
	Weight							
	Reps							
	Weight							

Cardio	Time	Distance	Heart Rate	Cals Burned

Measurements

Neck	R Bicep	L Bicep	Chest	Waist	Hips	R Thigh	L Thigh	Calf

Date:_____ Muscle Group: _____

S   M   T   W   T   F   S   Start Time_____
◯   ◯   ◯   ◯   ◯   ◯   ◯

Weight:_____   Finish Time_____

☐ Upper Body   ☐ Lower Body   ☐ Abs

Exercise	Set	1	2	3	4	5	6	7
	Reps							
	Weight							
	Reps							
	Weight							
	Reps							
	Weight							
	Reps							
	Weight							
	Reps							
	Weight							
	Reps							
	Weight							
	Reps							
	Weight							
	Reps							
	Weight							

Cardio	Time	Distance	Heart Rate	Cals Burned

Measurements

Neck	R Bicep	L Bicep	Chest	Waist	Hips	R Thigh	L Thigh	Calf

Date:_____ **Muscle Group:** _____

S M T W T F S   **Start Time**_____
◯ ◯ ◯ ◯ ◯ ◯ ◯

Weight:_____   **Finish Time**_____

☐ **Upper Body**   ☐ **Lower Body**   ☐ **Abs**

Exercise	Set	1	2	3	4	5	6	7
	Reps							
	Weight							
	Reps							
	Weight							
	Reps							
	Weight							
	Reps							
	Weight							
	Reps							
	Weight							
	Reps							
	Weight							
	Reps							
	Weight							
	Reps							
	Weight							

Cardio	Time	Distance	Heart Rate	Cals Burned

Measurements

Neck	R Bicep	L Bicep	Chest	Waist	Hips	R Thigh	L Thigh	Calf

Date:_____ **Muscle Group:** _____

S M T W T F S   **Start Time**_____
○ ○ ○ ○ ○ ○ ○

Weight:_____ **Finish Time**_____

☐ **Upper Body**   ☐ **Lower Body**   ☐ **Abs**

Exercise	Set	1	2	3	4	5	6	7
	Reps							
	Weight							
	Reps							
	Weight							
	Reps							
	Weight							
	Reps							
	Weight							
	Reps							
	Weight							
	Reps							
	Weight							
	Reps							
	Weight							
	Reps							
	Weight							

Cardio	Time	Distance	Heart Rate	Cals Burned

Measurements

Neck	R Bicep	L Bicep	Chest	Waist	Hips	R Thigh	L Thigh	Calf

Date:_____ **Muscle Group:** _____

S M T W T F S **Start Time**_____
◯ ◯ ◯ ◯ ◯ ◯ ◯

Weight:_____ **Finish Time**_____

☐ **Upper Body**   ☐ **Lower Body**   ☐ **Abs**

Exercise	Set	1	2	3	4	5	6	7
	Reps							
	Weight							
	Reps							
	Weight							
	Reps							
	Weight							
	Reps							
	Weight							
	Reps							
	Weight							
	Reps							
	Weight							
	Reps							
	Weight							
	Reps							
	Weight							

Cardio	Time	Distance	Heart Rate	Cals Burned

Measurements

Neck	R Bicep	L Bicep	Chest	Waist	Hips	R Thigh	L Thigh	Calf

Date:_____ Muscle Group: _____

S	M	T	W	T	F	S
○	○	○	○	○	○	○

Start Time_____

Weight:_____ Finish Time_____

☐ Upper Body   ☐ Lower Body   ☐ Abs

Exercise	Set	1	2	3	4	5	6	7
	Reps							
	Weight							
	Reps							
	Weight							
	Reps							
	Weight							
	Reps							
	Weight							
	Reps							
	Weight							
	Reps							
	Weight							
	Reps							
	Weight							
	Reps							
	Weight							

Cardio	Time	Distance	Heart Rate	Cals Burned

Measurements

Neck	R Bicep	L Bicep	Chest	Waist	Hips	R Thigh	L Thigh	Calf

Date:_____   Muscle Group: _____

S   M   T   W   T   F   S   Start Time_____
○   ○   ○   ○   ○   ○   ○

Weight:_____   Finish Time_____

☐ Upper Body   ☐ Lower Body   ☐ Abs

Exercise	Set	1	2	3	4	5	6	7
	Reps							
	Weight							
	Reps							
	Weight							
	Reps							
	Weight							
	Reps							
	Weight							
	Reps							
	Weight							
	Reps							
	Weight							
	Reps							
	Weight							
	Reps							
	Weight							

Cardio	Time	Distance	Heart Rate	Cals Burned

Measurements

Neck	R Bicep	L Bicep	Chest	Waist	Hips	R Thigh	L Thigh	Calf

Date:_____   Muscle Group: _____

S   M   T   W   T   F   S   Start Time_____
◯   ◯   ◯   ◯   ◯   ◯   ◯

Weight:_____   Finish Time_____

☐ Upper Body   ☐ Lower Body   ☐ Abs

Exercise	Set	1	2	3	4	5	6	7
	Reps							
	Weight							
	Reps							
	Weight							
	Reps							
	Weight							
	Reps							
	Weight							
	Reps							
	Weight							
	Reps							
	Weight							
	Reps							
	Weight							
	Reps							
	Weight							

Cardio	Time	Distance	Heart Rate	Cals Burned

Measurements

Neck	R Bicep	L Bicep	Chest	Waist	Hips	R Thigh	L Thigh	Calf

Date:_____ Muscle Group: _____

| S | M | T | W | T | F | S |
| ○ | ○ | ○ | ○ | ○ | ○ | ○ |

Start Time_____

Weight:_____ Finish Time_____

☐ Upper Body   ☐ Lower Body   ☐ Abs

Exercise	Set	1	2	3	4	5	6	7
	Reps							
	Weight							
	Reps							
	Weight							
	Reps							
	Weight							
	Reps							
	Weight							
	Reps							
	Weight							
	Reps							
	Weight							
	Reps							
	Weight							
	Reps							
	Weight							

Cardio	Time	Distance	Heart Rate	Cals Burned

Measurements

Neck	R Bicep	L Bicep	Chest	Waist	Hips	R Thigh	L Thigh	Calf

Date:_____ Muscle Group: _____

S   M   T   W   T   F   S   Start Time_____
◯ ◯ ◯ ◯ ◯ ◯ ◯

Weight:_____ Finish Time_____

☐ Upper Body   ☐ Lower Body   ☐ Abs

Exercise	Set	1	2	3	4	5	6	7
	Reps							
	Weight							
	Reps							
	Weight							
	Reps							
	Weight							
	Reps							
	Weight							
	Reps							
	Weight							
	Reps							
	Weight							
	Reps							
	Weight							
	Reps							
	Weight							

Cardio	Time	Distance	Heart Rate	Cals Burned

Measurements

Neck	R Bicep	L Bicep	Chest	Waist	Hips	R Thigh	L Thigh	Calf

Date:_____   **Muscle Group:** _____

S   M   T   W   T   F   S   **Start Time**_____
○   ○   ○   ○   ○   ○   ○

Weight:_____   **Finish Time**_____

☐ **Upper Body**   ☐ **Lower Body**   ☐ **Abs**

Exercise	Set	1	2	3	4	5	6	7
	Reps							
	Weight							
	Reps							
	Weight							
	Reps							
	Weight							
	Reps							
	Weight							
	Reps							
	Weight							
	Reps							
	Weight							
	Reps							
	Weight							
	Reps							
	Weight							

Cardio	Time	Distance	Heart Rate	Cals Burned

Measurements

Neck	R Bicep	L Bicep	Chest	Waist	Hips	R Thigh	L Thigh	Calf

Date:_____ Muscle Group: _____

S M T W T F S   Start Time_____
○ ○ ○ ○ ○ ○ ○

Weight:_____   Finish Time_____

☐ Upper Body   ☐ Lower Body   ☐ Abs

Exercise	Set	1	2	3	4	5	6	7
	Reps							
	Weight							
	Reps							
	Weight							
	Reps							
	Weight							
	Reps							
	Weight							
	Reps							
	Weight							
	Reps							
	Weight							
	Reps							
	Weight							
	Reps							
	Weight							

Cardio	Time	Distance	Heart Rate	Cals Burned

Measurements

Neck	R Bicep	L Bicep	Chest	Waist	Hips	R Thigh	L Thigh	Calf

Date:_____ Muscle Group: _____

S M T W T F S   Start Time_____
○ ○ ○ ○ ○ ○ ○

Weight:_____   Finish Time_____

☐ Upper Body   ☐ Lower Body   ☐ Abs

Exercise	Set	1	2	3	4	5	6	7
	Reps							
	Weight							
	Reps							
	Weight							
	Reps							
	Weight							
	Reps							
	Weight							
	Reps							
	Weight							
	Reps							
	Weight							
	Reps							
	Weight							
	Reps							
	Weight							

Cardio	Time	Distance	Heart Rate	Cals Burned

Measurements

Neck	R Bicep	L Bicep	Chest	Waist	Hips	R Thigh	L Thigh	Calf

Date:_____ Muscle Group: _____

S M T W T F S   Start Time_____
◯ ◯ ◯ ◯ ◯ ◯ ◯

Weight:_____   Finish Time_____

☐ Upper Body   ☐ Lower Body   ☐ Abs

Exercise	Set	1	2	3	4	5	6	7
	Reps							
	Weight							
	Reps							
	Weight							
	Reps							
	Weight							
	Reps							
	Weight							
	Reps							
	Weight							
	Reps							
	Weight							
	Reps							
	Weight							
	Reps							
	Weight							

Cardio	Time	Distance	Heart Rate	Cals Burned

Measurements

Neck	R Bicep	L Bicep	Chest	Waist	Hips	R Thigh	L Thigh	Calf

Date:_____   **Muscle Group:** _____

S   M   T   W   T   F   S   **Start Time**_____
◯ ◯ ◯ ◯ ◯ ◯ ◯

Weight:_____   **Finish Time**_____

☐ **Upper Body**   ☐ **Lower Body**   ☐ **Abs**

Exercise	Set	1	2	3	4	5	6	7
	Reps							
	Weight							
	Reps							
	Weight							
	Reps							
	Weight							
	Reps							
	Weight							
	Reps							
	Weight							
	Reps							
	Weight							
	Reps							
	Weight							
	Reps							
	Weight							

Cardio	Time	Distance	Heart Rate	Cals Burned

Measurements

Neck	R Bicep	L Bicep	Chest	Waist	Hips	R Thigh	L Thigh	Calf

Date:_____ **Muscle Group:** _____

S	M	T	W	T	F	S
○	○	○	○	○	○	○

Start Time_____

Weight:_____ **Finish Time**_____

☐ **Upper Body**   ☐ **Lower Body**   ☐ **Abs**

Exercise	Set	1	2	3	4	5	6	7
	Reps							
	Weight							
	Reps							
	Weight							
	Reps							
	Weight							
	Reps							
	Weight							
	Reps							
	Weight							
	Reps							
	Weight							
	Reps							
	Weight							
	Reps							
	Weight							

Cardio	Time	Distance	Heart Rate	Cals Burned

Measurements

Neck	R Bicep	L Bicep	Chest	Waist	Hips	R Thigh	L Thigh	Calf

Date:_____   Muscle Group: _____

S M T W T F S   Start Time_____
◯ ◯ ◯ ◯ ◯ ◯ ◯

Weight:_____   Finish Time_____

☐ Upper Body   ☐ Lower Body   ☐ Abs

Exercise	Set	1	2	3	4	5	6	7
	Reps							
	Weight							
	Reps							
	Weight							
	Reps							
	Weight							
	Reps							
	Weight							
	Reps							
	Weight							
	Reps							
	Weight							
	Reps							
	Weight							
	Reps							
	Weight							

Cardio	Time	Distance	Heart Rate	Cals Burned

Measurements

Neck	R Bicep	L Bicep	Chest	Waist	Hips	R Thigh	L Thigh	Calf

Date:_____ Muscle Group: _____

S M T W T F S   Start Time_____
◯ ◯ ◯ ◯ ◯ ◯ ◯

Weight:_____   Finish Time_____

☐ Upper Body   ☐ Lower Body   ☐ Abs

Exercise	Set	1	2	3	4	5	6	7
	Reps							
	Weight							
	Reps							
	Weight							
	Reps							
	Weight							
	Reps							
	Weight							
	Reps							
	Weight							
	Reps							
	Weight							
	Reps							
	Weight							
	Reps							
	Weight							

Cardio	Time	Distance	Heart Rate	Cals Burned

Measurements

Neck	R Bicep	L Bicep	Chest	Waist	Hips	R Thigh	L Thigh	Calf

Date:_____ **Muscle Group:** _____

S M T W T F S   **Start Time**_____
◯ ◯ ◯ ◯ ◯ ◯ ◯

Weight:_____   **Finish Time**_____

☐ **Upper Body**   ☐ **Lower Body**   ☐ **Abs**

Exercise	Set	1	2	3	4	5	6	7
	Reps							
	Weight							
	Reps							
	Weight							
	Reps							
	Weight							
	Reps							
	Weight							
	Reps							
	Weight							
	Reps							
	Weight							
	Reps							
	Weight							
	Reps							
	Weight							

Cardio	Time	Distance	Heart Rate	Cals Burned

Measurements

Neck	R Bicep	L Bicep	Chest	Waist	Hips	R Thigh	L Thigh	Calf

Date:_____ **Muscle Group:** _____

S M T W T F S **Start Time**_____
◯ ◯ ◯ ◯ ◯ ◯ ◯

Weight:_____ **Finish Time**_____

☐ **Upper Body**   ☐ **Lower Body**   ☐ **Abs**

Exercise	Set	1	2	3	4	5	6	7
	Reps							
	Weight							
	Reps							
	Weight							
	Reps							
	Weight							
	Reps							
	Weight							
	Reps							
	Weight							
	Reps							
	Weight							
	Reps							
	Weight							
	Reps							
	Weight							

Cardio	Time	Distance	Heart Rate	Cals Burned

Measurements

Neck	R Bicep	L Bicep	Chest	Waist	Hips	R Thigh	L Thigh	Calf

Date:_____ Muscle Group: _____

S M T W T F S   Start Time_____

◯ ◯ ◯ ◯ ◯ ◯ ◯

Weight:_____   Finish Time_____

☐ Upper Body   ☐ Lower Body   ☐ Abs

Exercise	Set	1	2	3	4	5	6	7
	Reps							
	Weight							
	Reps							
	Weight							
	Reps							
	Weight							
	Reps							
	Weight							
	Reps							
	Weight							
	Reps							
	Weight							
	Reps							
	Weight							
	Reps							
	Weight							

Cardio	Time	Distance	Heart Rate	Cals Burned

Measurements

Neck	R Bicep	L Bicep	Chest	Waist	Hips	R Thigh	L Thigh	Calf

Date:_____   **Muscle Group:** _____

S   M   T   W   T   F   S   **Start Time**_____
◯ ◯ ◯ ◯ ◯ ◯ ◯

Weight:_____   **Finish Time**_____

☐ **Upper Body**   ☐ **Lower Body**   ☐ **Abs**

Exercise	Set	1	2	3	4	5	6	7
	Reps							
	Weight							
	Reps							
	Weight							
	Reps							
	Weight							
	Reps							
	Weight							
	Reps							
	Weight							
	Reps							
	Weight							
	Reps							
	Weight							
	Reps							
	Weight							

Cardio	Time	Distance	Heart Rate	Cals Burned

Measurements

Neck	R Bicep	L Bicep	Chest	Waist	Hips	R Thigh	L Thigh	Calf

Date:_____ Muscle Group: _____

S	M	T	W	T	F	S
◯	◯	◯	◯	◯	◯	◯

Start Time_____

Weight:_____ Finish Time_____

☐ Upper Body   ☐ Lower Body   ☐ Abs

Exercise	Set	1	2	3	4	5	6	7
	Reps							
	Weight							
	Reps							
	Weight							
	Reps							
	Weight							
	Reps							
	Weight							
	Reps							
	Weight							
	Reps							
	Weight							
	Reps							
	Weight							
	Reps							
	Weight							

Cardio	Time	Distance	Heart Rate	Cals Burned

Measurements

Neck	R Bicep	L Bicep	Chest	Waist	Hips	R Thigh	L Thigh	Calf

Date:_____ **Muscle Group:** _____

S M T W T F S   **Start Time**_____
○ ○ ○ ○ ○ ○ ○

Weight:_____ **Finish Time**_____

☐ **Upper Body**   ☐ **Lower Body**   ☐ **Abs**

Exercise	Set	1	2	3	4	5	6	7
	Reps							
	Weight							
	Reps							
	Weight							
	Reps							
	Weight							
	Reps							
	Weight							
	Reps							
	Weight							
	Reps							
	Weight							
	Reps							
	Weight							
	Reps							
	Weight							

Cardio	Time	Distance	Heart Rate	Cals Burned

Measurements

Neck	R Bicep	L Bicep	Chest	Waist	Hips	R Thigh	L Thigh	Calf

Date:_____ **Muscle Group:** _____

S M T W T F S   **Start Time**_____
◯ ◯ ◯ ◯ ◯ ◯ ◯

Weight:_____ **Finish Time**_____

☐ **Upper Body**   ☐ **Lower Body**   ☐ **Abs**

Exercise	Set	1	2	3	4	5	6	7
	Reps							
	Weight							
	Reps							
	Weight							
	Reps							
	Weight							
	Reps							
	Weight							
	Reps							
	Weight							
	Reps							
	Weight							
	Reps							
	Weight							
	Reps							
	Weight							

Cardio	Time	Distance	Heart Rate	Cals Burned

Measurements

Neck	R Bicep	L Bicep	Chest	Waist	Hips	R Thigh	L Thigh	Calf

Thank you!

WE ARE GLAD THAT YOU PURCHASED OUR
BOOK!
PLEASE LET US KNOW HOW WE CAN IMPROVE IT!
YOUR FEEDBACK IS ESSENTIAL TO US.

Contact us at:

M   log'Sin@gmail.com

JUST TITLE THE EMAIL 'CREATIVE' AND WE WILL
GIVE YOU SOME EXTRA SURPRISES!

www.ingramcontent.com/pod-product-compliance
Lightning Source LLC
Chambersburg PA
CBHW070539030426
42337CB00016B/2267